OSTOMY DIET COOKBOOK

Delicious And Nutrient-Packed Friendly Recipes For Pretentious Nourishment And Vibrant Lifestyle

DR LUCAS KAYCE

DISCLAIMER

This book about illness and nutrition is not meant to replace expert medical advice, diagnosis, or treatment; rather, it is meant purely for informational reasons. This book's content is founded on broad concepts and recommendations for managing diseases and nutrition.

Before adopting any major dietary or lifestyle changes, readers are recommended to speak with a qualified healthcare provider, such as a licensed physician or registered dietitian, especially if they have pre-existing medical concerns. Everybody has different health demands, so what works for one person might not work for another.

The use of the information provided in this book may have unfavorable repercussions or consequences, for which the author and publisher disclaim all liability. No disease is meant to be identified, treated, cured, or prevented by the information provided.

The book may include contain references to medical literature or research findings; however readers are urged to independently confirm this material and contact reliable sources.

It is important to remember that the fields of nutrition and medicine are always changing, and that new findings could have an impact on the advice offered in this book. As a result, readers are urged to keep up with the most recent advancements in healthcare and, when in doubt, seek professional counsel.

By reading this book, readers agree that they are in charge of their own health decisions and release the author and publisher from any liability arising from the use of the material in the book, whether direct or indirect.

TABLE OF CONTENTS

ABOUT THE BOOK

For those navigating life after ostomy surgery, the "Ostomy Diet Cookbook" is an invaluable resource. Taking into account the particular dietary requirements of those who have an ostomy, this cookbook offers a wealth of ostomy-friendly dishes along with helpful advice. In addition to extending a hearty welcome, the introduction section explains ostomy and offers tips for using the cookbook efficiently.

The book covers the basics of ostomies, including information on the many kinds and practical advice for day-to-day living. The book "Nutrition and Ostomy" explains the importance of proteins, carbs, lipids, and water in promoting a well-balanced diet that aids in post-ostomy healing.

The cookbook then deftly moves into helpful guidance on what foods to eat—like fruits that are good for ostomies, lean proteins, and whole grains—while also emphasizing what foods to avoid since they may cause problems.

This cookbook stands out for its emphasis on ostomate-friendly cooking methods. Guidance on ostomy-safe cooking techniques, inventive flavor enhancement tactics, and meal preparation advice are provided to readers to guarantee a pleasurable and health-conscious culinary experience. The book also offers advice on how to adjust and modify well-loved dishes for an ostomy-friendly diet, along with dos and don'ts.

The book sample meal plans provide balanced options for weekday meals, quick dishes for hectic days, and menus for special occasions, catering to a wide range of dietary requirements. Snack suggestions are covered, which offers ostomy patients healthful ways to satiate appetites without compromising their health. The handbook also tackles the difficulty of eating out, providing helpful guidance on interpreting menus, explaining dietary requirements, and even keeping a balanced diet when traveling.

The cookbook goes outside the kitchen to investigate the relationship among food choices, physical exercise, and mental health. The book encourages a comprehensive approach to ostomy health by providing information on interacting with the ostomy community. All things considered, the "Ostomy Diet Cookbook" is a vital tool that enables people to adopt a happy and health-conscious lifestyle following ostomy surgery.

WELCOME TO COOKBOOK FOR THE OSTOMY DIET

Welcome to the Ostomy Diet Cookbook, an extensive resource designed to meet the specific dietary requirements of those who have an ostomy. There are many obstacles to overcome when managing life with an ostomy and sustaining general health depends in large part on careful diet planning. The goal of this cookbook is to enable people who have an ostomy to enjoy a healthy and fulfilling diet by offering helpful advice, delectable recipes, and insightful information.

COMPREHENDING DIETARY REQUIREMENTS AND OSTOMY

It is crucial to have a thorough grasp of ostomy and the related dietary issues before starting this culinary adventure. An ostomy is a surgical treatment that makes a hole in the body for waste to exit, rerouting the body's duties that were previously fulfilled by the natural organs. Colostomy, ileostomy, and urostomy are common forms of ostomies, each requiring unique adaptations and difficulties.

The digestive and absorption processes of people who have an ostomy frequently alter, which affects how the body absorbs and uses nutrients. It is critical to understand that each person's experience with an ostomy is distinct and that dietary requirements might change depending on the type of ostomy and the health of the individual. These subtleties are taken into consideration in this cookbook, which provides a wide variety of dishes that may be modified to meet various dietary choices, constraints, and nutritional needs.

It is essential to comprehend how ostomy and nutrition work together to preserve health and avoid issues. To properly manage symptoms, people may need to modify their eating habits as certain foods may have an impact on the regularity and consistency of their stools. For those who have an ostomy, maintaining digestive health and general well-being is greatly influenced by variables including hydration, fiber consumption, and the proper ratio of vital nutrients.

We'll go into more detail about specific dietary recommendations and the dos and don'ts of an ostomy-friendly diet in the cookbook's subsequent sections. With advice on everything from gas and odor management to cooking tasty and healthy foods, the Ostomy Diet Cookbook hopes to become a reliable friend that helps people embrace a happy and healthy lifestyle following ostomy surgery. Together, let's go on this culinary journey that will encourage enjoyment and empowerment in addition to nourishing food at each meal.

CHAPTER ONE

BASICS OF OSTOMY

WHAT IS AN OSTOMY?

An ostomy is a surgical operation in which the passage of bodily waste is directed through the creation of an abdominal orifice, or stoma. When a part of the digestive or urinary system needs to be bypassed or removed because of an illness, trauma, or congenital problem, this treatment is frequently required. Body waste, such as urine or stool, can leave the body through the stoma and gather in an external pouching system. Most often, ostomies are used to treat diseases including diverticulitis, inflammatory bowel illness, colorectal cancer, or congenital abnormalities that affect the urinary or gastrointestinal tract.

OSTOMY TYPES

Ostomies come in different varieties, each called after the organ they involve and the particular surgery that is done. Ileostomy, urostomy, and colostomy are the three main varieties. Diverting the colon to the abdominal surface is known as a colostomy, and it is frequently used to treat diseases including Crohn's disease and colorectal cancer.

An ileostomy, which is typically done to treat illnesses like ulcerative colitis, entails raising the ileum—the lowest portion of the small intestine—to the surface of the abdomen. In contrast, a urostomy entails rerouting urine from the bladder through a stoma and is typically required following bladder removal due to malignancy.

ADVICE AND TIPS FOR LIVING WITH AN OSTOMY

Although having an ostomy might cause mental and physical difficulties, people can have happy, fulfilled lives if they receive the right support and care. Knowing how to maintain the pouching system is essential to maintaining an ostomy.

Skin irritation and infection can be avoided with regular changes and good cleaning. It's critical to collaborate closely with medical professionals to identify the ideal pouch and accessories for a person's lifestyle and body type.

For those who have an ostomy, emotional and psychological well-being are just as vital as physical care. It might be quite helpful to join support groups, get counseling, or connect with people who have experienced similar things. An atmosphere of support can be established by open communication with friends, family, and healthcare professionals. While it may take some time to develop a good body image and sense of self, accepting one's new circumstances and putting an emphasis on general health and wellness can help one adopt a positive outlook.

Living with an ostomy frequently involves adjusting to a new food and way of life. Many find that they can have a varied and satisfying diet, even though there may be some dietary restrictions. Drinking enough water, adding fiber gradually, and keeping an eye on personal tolerances can all help create a balanced and healthful diet. In addition, regular physical activity is advised, taking into account personal fitness levels and any advice from medical professionals.

An ostomy is a surgical technique that makes an incision in the abdomen to reroute waste products from the body. Common ostomy kinds include ileostomy, urostomy, and colostomy, each of which treats a particular medical issue. Managing an ostomy involves both medical and psychological support. Effectively navigating life with an ostomy requires knowledge of and skill with the pouching system, finding support, and adjusting to changes in lifestyle. Following ostomy surgery, people can have happy, busy lives if they have access to the appropriate resources and adopt a positive outlook.

CHAPTER TWO

OSTOMY AND NUTRITION

NUTRITION IS IMPORTANT AFTER OSTOMY SURGERY

A person's general health and recuperation following ostomy surgery are greatly influenced by their diet. It is impossible to exaggerate how crucial nutrition is after ostomy surgery because it has a direct impact on both physical health and overall quality of life.

People, who have an ostomy, or ostomates, frequently deal with particular issues that need careful consideration while making food decisions to maintain adequate nutrition.

The need to balance important nutrients is one of the most important factors in a post-ostomy diet. The three basic macronutrients—proteins, carbs, and fats—each have unique functions within the body. Proteins are essential for muscle preservation and tissue repair, which is especially crucial for ostomates during their recuperation. A person's main energy source, carbohydrates aids in the restoration of strength and stamina. Good fats promote skin health and help absorb fat-soluble vitamins, which are critical for overall health.

MAINTAINING A HEALTHY BALANCE OF PROTEINS, CARBOHYDRATES, AND FATS

Meal planning needs to be planned carefully and comprehensively to balance these nutrients. To promote muscular function and repair, ostomates should give priority to foods high in lean proteins, such as fish, poultry, and tofu. Including complex carbs from fruits, vegetables, and whole grains helps sustain energy levels without aggravating the digestive system. Furthermore, incorporating wholesome fats from foods like nuts, avocados, and olive oil can enhance the nutritional value and well-roundedness of a diet.

For ostomates, enough hydration is just as important as macronutrients. It's critical to keep drinking enough water to avoid dehydration, which can be a common worry after ostomy surgery. Osteomates may be more susceptible to dehydration because of variations in the digestive system's ability to absorb fluids. As a result, maintaining adequate hydration is crucial for good health in general and can help avoid issues like electrolyte imbalances.

TIPS FOR HYDRATION FOR OSTOMATES

Ostomates should drink small amounts of water throughout the day instead of consuming big amounts at once. This will assist control of fluid absorption and reduce the possibility of excessively watery ostomy output. Selecting foods that are high in water and nutrients, such as fruits and vegetables, is a good idea. Urine color can be used as a straightforward indicator of one's level of hydration; in general, a pale yellow tint indicates adequate hydration.

A post-ostomy diet is a vital component of healing and continuous health maintenance for ostomy patients. Maintaining a balance of vital nutrients, such as lipids, proteins, and carbs, encourages recovery and enhances general health. Equally crucial is hydration, and sodomites should take precautions to keep their fluid balance in check. Ostomates can improve their recovery, control potential complications, and lead meaningful and healthy lives by carefully monitoring their diet and fluid consumption.

CHAPTER THREE

FOODS TO ACCEPT

SUITABLE FRUITS AND VEGETABLES FOR OSTOMIES

For those who have an ostomy, eating a healthy, well-balanced diet is essential, and including ostomy-friendly fruits and vegetables is vital to preserving general health. Choosing foods that are simple to digest can reduce the possibility of discomfort or other issues.

For example, bananas are a favorite fruit since they are easy on the stomach and high in vital nutrients. Another great option is cooked and peeled apples, which provide dietary fiber without the risk of skin irritation from raw fruit.

When it comes to vegetables, cooked carrots, and zucchini are generally well-tolerated and a good source of vitamins and minerals. Easier to digest, steamed spinach or kale can add to a diet rich in nutrients. Tolerances might vary, so people with ostomies must try a variety of fruits and vegetables to see which ones work best for their digestive systems.

SKELETAL MUSCLE FOR OSTOMY HEALTH

Lean proteins help with tissue regeneration and maintenance, thus including them in the diet is essential for maintaining good ostomy health. Choosing easily digested protein sources can help avert issues and discomfort.

Lean fish cuts and skinless poultry, such as chicken or turkey, are great options. In addition to being higher in vital amino acids, these proteins also tend to be kinder to the digestive tract.

Tofu and legumes like lentils and chickpeas can be a useful source of protein for plant-based eaters or vegetarians. Cooking these items to a high temperature will improve their digestion. Meal planning and portion control are crucial for ensuring a well-balanced protein intake while minimizing undue stress on the digestive system.

WHOLE GRAINS AND HANDLING FIBER

For those who have an ostomy, whole grains are an important part of a balanced diet because they provide vital minerals and dietary fiber.

However, controlling fiber intake is essential to avoiding potential problems like clogs. It is possible to add whole grains like quinoa, brown rice, and oats to the diet, but it is crucial to do so gradually and monitor the body's reaction.

Certain high-fiber meals may need to be avoided by some people, or if whole grains are difficult for them to digest, they may need to switch to refined grains. Digestion of grains can be facilitated by fully cooking them and drinking plenty of water.

Incorporating soluble fiber—which comes from foods like applesauce, bananas, and oatmeal—can also be advantageous because it is generally easier on the digestive tract than insoluble fiber, which is present in some vegetables and entire grains.

Adopting ostomy-friendly fruits and vegetables, lean proteins, and controlling whole grain and fiber consumption all require a customized strategy. To ensure adequate nutrition and general well-being, people should collaborate closely with healthcare providers and nutritionists to customize their diets to meet their unique needs.

CHAPTER FOUR

FOODS AT HIGH RISK FOR OSTOMATES

People, who have ostomies, whether as a result of surgery or illnesses like Crohn's disease or colorectal cancer, frequently have to watch what they eat. Ostomates may experience discomfort, obstructions, or other difficulties as a result of certain diets. High-fiber foods can be problematic for people with ostomies because they can be difficult to digest and can cause bowel blockages. This is especially true of foods with tough skins or seeds.

Broccoli, cabbage, and cauliflower are examples of cruciferous vegetables that are under observation for ostomates. Despite their high fiber content and propensity to induce gas, these veggies are rich in nutrients and may be uncomfortable for people who have an ostomy. Furthermore, meals that are heavy in fat and/or spicy may cause irritation or inflammation around the stoma, so these foods are not as recommended for people who have this problem.

MAKING WISE FOOD SELECTIONS TO CONTROL GAS AND ODOR

Gas and odor generation are major issues for ostomates, as they can pose social challenges and negatively affect their confidence. Making thoughtful dietary choices that reduce gas production and prevent odor is crucial to addressing this. Limiting the consumption of foods that cause gas, such as beans, lentils, and carbonated drinks, may be advantageous for ostomates. These foods may increase the amount of gas in the digestive tract, which may cause discomfort and a visible odor.

Gum chewing and some sugar-free goods with sorbitol or mannitol may also cause gas production. Ostomates should think about using other sweeteners instead of artificial sweeteners, which might cause digestive problems if consumed in excess. Furthermore, being well hydrated is essential since it can facilitate easier digestion and help avoid constipation, which lowers the risk of problems associated with gas.

FOODS THAT COULD IRRITATE YOUR SKIN

For ostomates, some foods may irritate the region surrounding their stoma, which can be painful and potentially create difficulties if not taken care of properly. Acidic fruits, spicy foods, and drinks like citrus juices can irritate the stoma and the skin around it. Ostomates should limit their consumption of these meals and monitor their body's reaction.

In addition, foods that are scratchy or coarse, such as nuts and seeds, can irritate the skin and create pain for ostomy patients. Additionally, there's a chance that certain foods could clog digestive tracts.

 Ostomates must be careful with their diet, observing the texture and makeup of the items they eat and making necessary alterations to reduce the possibility of irritation and problems.

To maintain comfort and avoid difficulties, people with ostomies must be careful about the foods they eat. Ostomates who are aware of the possible hazards connected to specific foods—especially those that are high in fiber, cause gas or irritate the stomach—can make well-informed choices that will improve their general health and quality of life.

CHAPTER FIVE

COOKING METHODS

RECIPES SAFE FOR OSTOMIES

Cooking for someone who has an ostomy requires you to use techniques that put their digestive health first. It is advised to use steaming since it makes food soft without using a lot of fats or oils. This technique facilitates better digestion without sacrificing the products' nutritional value. Another ostomy-safe cooking technique that works well for veggies and lean proteins is boiling. The ease of boiling guarantees that little in the way of additives is required, preserving the dish's integrity without sacrificing the comfort of the digestive tract.

Baking is a flexible and ostomy-friendly method that may be used to make a range of foods with regulated fat content. Additionally, it gives food a nice texture without requiring a lot of flavor. Grilling is a good method for roommates who enjoy a little smoked flavor in their food. Grilled food can be tasty and easily digested by eschewing thick marinades and choosing for milder flavors.

INNOVATIVE TECHNIQUES FOR INCREASING FLAVOR WITHOUT AFFECTING DIGESTION

Herbs and spices become invaluable partners for ostomates who want to enhance the flavor of their meals without compromising digestion. Fresh herbs like parsley, cilantro, and basil give a visually pleasing presentation in addition to adding bright flavors. You may add a burst of freshness without using heavy sauces by using citrus zest or juice. Dressings on a mustard or vinegar basis are great ways to bring tart flavors to salads or protein dishes without adding too much fat.

Use aromatic items in moderation, such as ginger and garlic, to add depth of flavor. Vegetables' inherent sweetness can be enhanced by roasting them with a little olive oil, all without adding too much fat. Trying out various herb-infused oils or flavored vinegar can also give meals a distinctive twist without sacrificing ease of digestion.

ADVICE ON MEAL PREPARATION FOR COUPLES

For those who have an ostomy, efficient meal preparation is essential to a hassle-free and pleasurable dining experience. On days when you might not feel like cooking, batch cooking, and portion freezing might save you time and effort. Vegetables may be assembled quickly and easily during mealtime by precutting them and storing them in portion-sized containers, which eliminates the need for lengthy chopping and preparation.

For ostomates, incorporating a range of textures into meals can improve their entire dining experience. To ensure a comfortable dining experience, using appliances like blenders or food processors can assist generate smooth purees or finely chopped items. It's important to plan nutrient-dense meals while keeping in mind potential intestinal triggers.

Maintaining a meal journal can be beneficial in monitoring personal reactions to various substances, assisting in recognizing and averting any discomfort.

Using ostomy-safe cooking techniques, coming up with inventive ways to add taste, and putting useful meal prep advice into practice all help people with ostomies have a great culinary experience that supports their digestive comfort and nutritional well-being.

CHAPTER SIX

RECIPE ADJUSTMENTS AND REPLACEMENTS

MODIFYING WELL-LOVED RECIPES TO SUIT OSTOMY NEEDS

When it comes to converting beloved recipes into ostomy-friendly meals, people with ostomies frequently confront particular difficulties that call for careful adjustments. Ostomy surgery entails cutting a hole in the abdomen to reroute the body's waste flow, which may affect food preferences. It's critical to concentrate on using products and cooking methods that provide tasty and nourishing meals while still being easy on the digestive system.

Selecting easily digestible foods is important when adjusting recipes for ostomy-friendly diets. Minimizing stress on the digestive tract can be achieved by choosing easily digested cereals, lean proteins, and well-cooked vegetables.

Furthermore, it may be advantageous to have lower-fiber foods because high-fiber foods may be more difficult for ostomates to digest.

The food's consistency is an additional factor to take into account. It is possible to alter recipes to produce smoother textures, which people with ostomies may find more comfortable to eat. Using finely ground meats, pureeing or mashing vegetables, and choosing softer grains are all good ways to get a smoother consistency without sacrificing flavor.

OSTOMY HEALTH INGREDIENT SUBSTITUTIONS

It is essential to choose suitable ingredient replacements to preserve ostomy health and still enjoy a wide range of flavors. People with ostomies should be aware of foods that could irritate their ostomies or produce gas or odor while modifying recipes. For example, switching to softer veggies like carrots or zucchini in place of some cruciferous vegetables can help lower the chance of discomfort.

Lean meats and fish that are quickly digested are often well-tolerated when it comes to protein sources. But for some who find meat difficult, adding other protein sources like tofu, eggs, or lentils can work well in its place. Experimentation is key to finding the right ingredients for each person's tolerances and preferences.

Dairy alternatives should be taken into account because some ostomates may have lactose intolerance or be sensitive to specific dairy products. Making the switch to plant-based or lactose-free options can still deliver the essential nutrients without causing problems with digestion. Consuming meals high in probiotics can also improve digestion and support a healthy gut.

TIPS & ADVICE FOR CHANGING RECIPES

When modifying recipes to accommodate ostomy-friendly diets, there are a few things to remember to do and not do. On the plus side, you may produce tasty and readily digestible recipes by experimenting with different cooking techniques like poaching, baking, or steaming.

It is recommended to use herbs and spices for seasoning because they enhance flavor without making digestion uncomfortable.

With some components, you must use caution nevertheless. Steer clear of high-fiber meals, seeds, and nuts in excess as these can cause digestive tract blockages. Reducing the amount of spicy or highly seasoned foods you eat can also assist avoid pain and irritability?

Dos include drinking enough water, since maintaining adequate hydration is essential for ostomy patients to preserve general health and avoid dehydration. When experimenting with new recipes, remember to listen to your body and notice any discomfort or unfavorable reactions. Personalized food recommendations for ostomy health can be greatly aided by routine consultation with medical professionals.

CHAPTER SEVEN

EXAMPLE MENUS
SUFFICIENT MEAL PLANS FOR VARIOUS DIETARY REQUIREMENTS:

Developing well-rounded meal plans that accommodate different dietary requirements is essential to fostering general health and well-being. Whether people eat omnivorously, paleo, vegan, or vegetarian, a well-balanced diet guarantees that they get the right amounts of vital vitamins, minerals, and other nutrients. Vegans and vegetarians must include a range of plant-based protein sources, such as quinoa, tofu, and lentils. To attain balance, omnivores can concentrate on a combination of lean proteins, whole grains, and veggies.

When creating these meal plans, balancing macronutrients—proteins, carbs, and fats—is essential. Every macronutrient has a specific role, and when they are combined in the right way, they can boost muscle growth, energy levels, and general wellness. To maximize the amount of nutrients available while reducing the amount of processed foods and added sugars, whole foods—such as fruits, vegetables, whole grains, and lean proteins—are given priority.

Meal plan customization also entails taking dietary limitations and personal preferences into account. Some people might need gluten-free choices; others might need to watch how much sodium they eat. These variables are taken into consideration by a well-balanced meal plan, which guarantees that people can follow their dietary preferences without sacrificing their nutritional requirements. In general, for example, meal plans should emphasize flexibility, diversity, and balance to accommodate a range of dietary preferences.

OSTOMY-FRIENDLY FAST AND SIMPLE RECIPES FOR BUSY DAYS

Those who have an ostomy may find it difficult to manage their meals on hectic days, but it is possible with the correct quick and simple recipes. Ostomy-friendly recipes emphasize simple-to-digest items that are easy on the digestive tract, allowing people to be comfortable and avoid problems. These recipes frequently call for soft-textured meals including properly cooked veggies, lean meats, and easily digested grains.

It is essential to include a range of flavors and textures in ostomy-friendly meals to keep them appealing. For instance, quinoa and steamed veggies paired with grilled chicken or fish can make for a well-balanced, easily digestible meal.

Furthermore, those with ostomies may find it easier to handle modest, frequent meals throughout the day, which can assist in minimizing discomfort and controlling energy levels.

Another important factor to consider on hectic days is portability. Easy-to-pack ostomy-friendly dishes, such as salads with lean protein and soft fruits, help people stay on track with a balanced diet even when they're on the go. Drinking plenty of water is just as vital, and eating foods high in water content, such as cucumber and watermelon, can improve general health.

MENUS FOR SPECIAL OCCASIONS FOR OSTOMATES

Individuals with an ostomy can enjoy these events with carefully selected options that promote comfort and ease of digestion. Special occasions typically call for distinctive meals. It is crucial to concentrate on meals that are less prone to induce gas, bloating, or irritation when creating menus for special occasions for ostomates. Vegetables that are prepared to perfection, succulent meats, and readily absorbed carbohydrates can all be highlighted.

On special events, attention to portion sizes and timing is especially important. Meals that are smaller and more frequent throughout the event can assist ostomy patients manage their comfort level and avoid future problems. Having a wide selection of dishes enables personalization, meeting dietary requirements, and individual preferences.

Classic recipes can be made ostomy-friendly by using inventive ingredient substitutions in place of standard ones. For example, mashed sweet potatoes make a tasty and readily digestible substitute for mashed potatoes with a heavy cream base. For dessert, consider light, homemade sorbets or fruit-based delights to sate sweet appetites without jeopardizing intestinal comfort.

Ostomates' special occasion menus emphasize mild and easily digestible foods so that people may completely enjoy special occasions without worrying about their digestive health.

CHAPTER EIGHT

IDEAS FOR SNACKS

OSTOMATES' HEALTHY AND FILLING SNACKS

For those with ostomies, eating a healthy, balanced diet is essential since it supports general health and helps control any issues. Selecting snacks that are not only delicious but also easy on the digestive system is essential. Snacks that are high in nutrients, minimal in possible irritants, and simple to digest are beneficial for osteomates.

Fresh fruit is a wonderful option for ostomates. They offer fiber, vitamins, and minerals that are necessary without upsetting the stomach. Selecting softer fruits, such as melons, avocados, and bananas, can be especially kind to the digestive tract.

Yogurt also has probiotics that help intestinal health and is generally well-tolerated by ostomates, so adding it to snacks can be advantageous.

Snacks made of vegetables are yet another wholesome choice. Carrots, cucumbers, and bell peppers are examples of raw or minimally cooked veggies that have a delightful crunch and are packed full of vitamins. Combining them with hummus or a light dip can improve the snack's nutritional value and taste.

Lean protein sources like boiled eggs, grilled chicken, or turkey slices can be great options for anyone seeking an increase in protein.

These high-protein snacks provide sustained energy levels throughout the day and help promote feelings of fullness. Prioritizing lean proteins is crucial to prevent undue stress on the digestive system.

For ostomates, adding whole grains to snacks is also a wise decision. A little portion of quinoa, rice cakes, or whole-grain crackers can all be good sources of fiber that support regular digestion. But it's important to keep an eye on individual tolerances and select whole grains that the digestive system can easily process.

OPTIONS FOR CARRY-ALONG SNACKS FOR ACTIVE LIFESTYLES

Finding snacks that are both convenient and meet their nutritional needs can be a game-changer for people who lead hectic, mobile lives. For people who are constantly on the go, portable snacks are crucial because they give them access to wholesome meals all day long.

Because they are high in nutrients and good fats, nuts and seeds are great as on-the-go snacks. Nuts like chia seeds, walnuts, and almonds are easy to transport and provide you with a quick energy boost. Mixing nuts, seeds, and dried fruits to make a trail mix can be a delicious and filling snack choice.

A common option for busy people is a snack bar. Choose bars that are low in sugar and high in protein and fiber, especially those made with health-conscious consumers in mind. Making sure the bars you've selected fit your dietary needs and limits requires carefully reading the labeling.

Fresh fruit is an easy and convenient option, in addition to being healthful. Berries, bananas, and apples are simple to carry and need no preparation. Choosing pre-packaged fruit cups or chopping fruits into bite-sized pieces ahead of time might improve convenience without sacrificing nutritious content.

Single-serving containers of Greek yogurt are a great on-the-go snack since they provide a portable source of probiotics and protein. Try adding some granola or fresh fruit for variation. If you need to keep snacks cool during the day, you can store these yogurt cups in a cooler bag.

HEALTHY SNACKING PRACTICES FOR OSTOMIES

Ostomates have particular difficulties in keeping up a balanced, healthful diet, thus developing smart eating habits is crucial to their general wellbeing. When making snack plans, people should take into account a few important factors to promote the health of their ostomy.

An essential component of ostomy wellness is mindful eating. Chewing food well and savoring each bite can lessen the likelihood of blockages and decrease discomfort in the digestive system. Furthermore, it's critical to maintain hydration since it supports healthy digestion in general and facilitates digestion.

Snacking with minimal residue is another important tactic. Easy-to-digest foods with little fiber can reduce the likelihood of irritability and obstructions. Lean proteins, cooked and peeled veggies, and cooked grains are often well-tolerated and offer good snack options.

Ostomy health is significantly impacted by portion control. It can be easier to control digestion load and avoid pain if you eat smaller, more frequent meals and snacks throughout the day as opposed to a few big ones. Better digestion and nutrient absorption can be achieved by paying attention to portion amounts.

To identify trigger foods or products that may induce digestive troubles, ostomates can experiment with different foods and keep a food log. Through the process of monitoring their food choices and the symptoms that accompany them, people are better equipped to decide which snacks are appropriate for their particular needs.

It should be noted that intelligent snacking is essential for ostomates. Through the selection of nutrient-dense snacks, consideration of portability for people who lead busy lives, and use of ostomy health-promoting tactics, people can savor delightful snacks that enhance their general health.

CHAPTER NINE

EATING OUT WITH SELF-ASSURANCE

GETTING AROUND RESTAURANT MENUS

One of the first hurdles of dining out confidently is properly navigating restaurant menus. Searching the menu for terms that describe the ingredients and cooking techniques is essential. This can reveal information about how healthful the food is overall. Choosing baked, steamed, or grilled foods typically means they have been prepared less heavily than fried or sautéed foods. A well-balanced meal can also be achieved by watching portion sizes and taking into account the proportions of vegetables, proteins, and carbs.

Examining different menu items, like appetizers or side dishes, might also offer chances to tailor a meal to meet particular dietary requirements or tastes. A lot of restaurants are open to requests for changes, such as changing the ingredients or the way something is cooked. To guarantee a satisfying eating experience, it is crucial to express these preferences to the wait staff clearly and concisely.

INFORMING WAITSTAFF OF DIETARY REQUIREMENTS

When dining out, it's important to communicate your dietary requirements to the wait staff clearly and concisely. Expressing certain needs, such as dietary restrictions, intolerances, or preferences, in an aggressive yet kind manner enables the wait staff to comprehend and properly attend to such demands. Never be afraid to ask questions if you have any doubts about how to prepare a given cuisine. To guarantee client happiness, reputable eateries are frequently happy to share knowledge regarding ingredients and cooking techniques.

In certain situations, it could be advantageous to let the restaurant know ahead of time about any dietary requirements so they can make the appropriate arrangements.

Building a relationship with the wait staff can also improve the eating experience because they can make tailored suggestions or recommend appropriate dishes. Recall that effective communication encourages cooperation between the customer and the restaurant staff, creating a welcoming and upbeat environment.

MANAGING YOUR DIET AND TRAVELING WITH AN OSTOMY

When traveling with an ostomy, it takes extra thought and preparation to maintain a tasty and healthful meal. Finding eateries that are ostomy-friendly, have accessible facilities, and are prepared to make special accommodations is crucial. Tell the restaurant about your unique needs when making a reservation, including the necessity for a private restroom and disposal facilities.

When traveling, having backup ostomy supplies in addition to other necessities might provide one a sense of security. It's important to stay hydrated, so always have a bottle of water with you. Choose meals that are low in fiber and readily digested to reduce the chance of discomfort. Openly discuss your condition with the restaurant staff so they are aware of your needs and can make appropriate menu adjustments or suggestions.

Confidently dining out entails perusing menus with skill, informing wait staff of dietary requirements, and making sure that traveling with an ostomy is a flawless experience. People can savor a wide variety of gastronomic experiences without sacrificing their health or well-being by grasping these ideas.

CHAPTER TEN

OUTSIDE THE KITCHEN

ACTIVITY LEVELS AND OSTOMY HEALTH

Regular physical exercise is crucial for preserving general health, and this is also true for people who have an ostomy. For people who have ostomies, the idea of engaging in physical activity may seem overwhelming, but it's important to realize that having a stoma shouldn't stop you from living an active lifestyle. Under the right supervision, medical practitioners can assist people in finding hobbies and exercises that are appropriate for their particular situation.

It's important to adjust workout regimens to one's comfort level and pay heed to bodily signals. Walking, swimming, and yoga are examples of low-impact exercises that are frequently advised since they offer mildly effective ways to stay active without placing undue strain on the abdominal region.

Exercises that focus on strength training can also help to maintain muscular tone, which improves general physical health.

EMOTIONAL HEALTH AND NUTRITIONAL DECISIONS

There is a complex and frequently overlooked relationship between dietary choices and emotional well-being. The psychological effects of having a stoma can have a major impact on how people with ostomies relate to food. To promote a happy outlook, it's critical to recognize and deal with the emotional components of food decisions.

Eating a diet rich in nutrients and well-balanced is essential for good health and can also improve emotional stability. Maintaining energy levels and assisting the body's healing process are two important functions of nutrition. Healthcare providers can offer tailored advice on dietary decisions that complement a person's unique health requirements, guaranteeing optimal nutrition while taking into account any ostomy-related dietary restrictions.

MAKING SENSE OF THE OSTOMY COMMUNITY

Although having an ostomy can occasionally be a lonely experience, getting involved in the ostomy community can offer priceless support and inspiration. Building relationships with people who have gone through similar things can be empowering even outside of the kitchen. Online and offline support groups provide a forum for ostomy patients to exchange knowledge, counsel, and emotional support.

These groups offer a forum for people to talk about difficulties, acknowledge accomplishments, and share advice on coping with different ostomy-related issues. Making relationships with other ostomates not only offers useful information but also aids in overcoming feelings of loneliness. The ostomy community's common experiences can foster a spirit of resilience and camaraderie by serving as a constant reminder to individuals that they are not traveling this path alone.

Ostomy patients can prioritize physical activity for their general health, make thoughtful food choices to support their emotional well-being and connect with the ostomy community for understanding and support outside of the kitchen. Together, these elements support a comprehensive strategy for accepting and thriving in life following ostomy surgery.